EAT MORE AND LOSE WEIGHT:

KEEPING FIT NATURALY

Peter Wright

Copyright © Peter Wright, 2018

Disclaimer

All erudition contained in this book is given for informational and educational purposes only. The author is not in any way accountable for any results or outcomes that emanate from using this material. Constructive attempts have been made to provide information that is both accurate and effective, but the author is not bound for the accuracy or use/misuse of this information.

Contents

INTRODUCTION

The human body is biological machinery, and like every functional machinery, it is capable of wear and tear. A lack of proper care and maintenance of the human body will eventually lead to a collapse, as the body ages with time, and time reveals the body's weakness. This is why nowadays, individuals are very wary of their body fitness and health. A younger body is still well capable of enduring the mental and physical abuse thrown at it, but there is every tendency that the same lack of care for the body will begin to make a telling difference as an individual age. This, coupled with the increased pronunciation of the importance of fitness and how it impacts every area of our life has tilted the attention of the average individual towards his body health and fitness. The importance of being fit cannot be overemphasized.

Being fit makes us more energetic, reduces the risks of diseases and illness, thereby helping to save unnecessary medical expenses, boosts the chances of a longer life, promotes the mental health, increases self-confidence because of the feeling of being in control of my body, and will ultimately affect your quality of human relationship.

CHAPTER ONE

SETTING OUT

Setting out has to do with you determining how you desire your body to be. This is the first and one of the essential steps to building a fit and healthy body. You must firstly have a clear mental picture of the body physique you desire, as this will help you to determine the effort and sacrifice needed to get the desired results. Breaking the psychological barrier is a prerequisite to successfully achieving your body goals, as it is what will eventually sustain you through the unfamiliar territories that discipline will have to take you through. Draw out a clearly mapped plan, which is realistic and sustainable enough in the long term, and that will enhance the achievement of the preset goals. The plan will include details on your diet, and your daily routine, your dietary do's and don'ts, and finally, the expected body goal to keep you motivated all the way. In this way, working according to a plan will be made easier, as the necessary drive and motivation to abide by the designed system will not be lacking. While devising a result-oriented fitness plan that works for you, it is vital that you consider your age, free time, set goals, diet, biology, etc. Adherence to the plan religiously is very pivotal in achieving the desired results, and it will be a bonus if the plan can eventually be incorporated into your lifestyle, as it will ensure the longevity of the desired results.

CHAPTER TWO

DIET FOR A FIT AND HEALTHY BODY

Proper nutrition and a healthy lifestyle cannot be separated. Research has proven that an unhealthy diet and poor eating habit accounts for a majority of the health risks that people experience, and sometimes even death. Heart disease, hypertension, diabetes, obesity, and even cancer are all preventable, if only we make smart food choices every day. Since maintaining a healthy diet is an essential prerequisite to a healthy life, eating the right food at the right time will help supply the right calories and nutrients needed to develop and maintain a fit and healthy body capable of executing your day to day activities.

In order to develop a healthy and fit body, it is highly imperative that you know the exact food that supplies you with the nutrients and energy you require, while not simultaneously increasing your body fat levels. This will help you discover the food that will have a detrimental impact on your body fitness, and inform your decision on foods that feels right even though it is at the detriment of your health.

A healthy balanced diet consumed consistently is the fuel of a healthy and fit body. You should consume the right proportion of carbohydrates, proteins and other nutrients necessary for a fit and healthy body system before you then begin to think about an exercise routine to help keep your body in shape. The following nutrients are recommended for a fit and healthy body:

1) **Carbohydrate:** There is a popular notion that carbohydrate has to be excluded from your diet if you are going to maintain your body fitness. While this is true to a degree, it is not necessarily the healthiest eating strategy, especially if you work out regularly. This is because carbohydrates are the leading supplier of the energy the body needs to perform, so an outright removal of carbohydrate

from your diet is not sustainable in the long term. Preferably, a better alternative is to consume the right type of carbohydrate in the right quantity and at the right time. Instead of relying on simple carbohydrate found in sweet and processed food, you should redirect your focus towards complex carbohydrate that can be derived from fruits, vegetables, and whole grains. This sort of carbohydrate requires a longer time to be broken down into glucose. The body changes the carbohydrate into glucose, which is stored in the muscle as glycogen. As you exercise, the glycogen is finally transformed into energy needed to keep your body functioning at its maximum level. Also, endeavor to consume your carbohydrate earlier in the day as it gives more time for the carbohydrate to be converted into energy and be used up during the day rather than being stored as fats if it is not used up.

2) **PROTEIN:** Protein does not supply the energy needed to perform, but it is necessary for muscle

functioning. It helps the body in the growth, maintenance, and repair of muscles, and can even be a source of energy in the event of unavailability of carbohydrate. Protein can be gotten from animal and plant sources. Animal sources include chicken and turkey meat, beef, pork, fish, milk, and eggs. Plant sources, on the other hand, include beans, nuts, soy products, and seafood.

Even though the importance of protein for a healthy and fit body cannot be overemphasized, it is of equal importance that the intake of protein is not too much, as it capable of putting pressure on your kidney, and cause damage to the kidney. Hence, it is essential that you have an idea of the quantity of protein your body needs before consuming protein.

3) **FATS:** Consumption of the right proportion of Fats has been proven to be of immense importance in building a healthy body and mind. Just ensure that the proper type of Fats (unsaturated) is consumed, and make sure you achieve a balance between the

amount calories you consume and the number of calories you burn.

Healthy and unsaturated fats are essential in a healthy diet as it helps in the provision of the fatty acids and calories that are essential to keeping your body functioning, helps strengthen the immune system, boost the operation of the brain and nervous system, improve the function of organs and glands, boost energy and performance levels, help to reduce inflammation, and help to regulate body weight. Healthy and unsaturated fats can be gotten from foods like nuts, olives, avocado, vegetable oils, and fish such as salmon and tuna.

CHAPTER THREE

How to Balance Between Plant and Animal Protein

The muscles and organs of the body are made up of protein. Nearly all the processes that occur in your body are made possible because of protein. Protein is responsible for the building, repairing and maintenance of the structure of the body, and can be gotten from two sources namely plant and animal sources.

One of the significant differences between plant and animal protein is their amino acid content. The total number of essential or non-essential amino acids the body needs to build proteins is around 20 in number. However, the body is only able to produce the non-essential amino acids, so you have no choice than to source for the essential amino acids through your everyday diet.

Even though some people have claimed the protein source, be it plant, or animal shouldn't matter, others have stated that attention should be given to the source of the protein because of the difference in the amino acid content in the different protein sources, and also the rate of absorption of the amino acid by the body system. Animal protein is very similar to the type of protein contained in the human body. Hence it is absorbed and used up faster than the protein found in plants. Animal protein also essentially contains the greater quantity of amino acids that are needed by the body to function effectively as compared with plant protein. Majority of plant protein is inadequate, always lacking at least one essential amino acid. This has made it imperative that a balance is struck between the consumption of protein from plant and animal sources in such a way that no essential amino acid will be missed out on.

Whenever you are faced with the task of deciding the balance between the intake of plant or animal protein, it is essential that you consider the wide nutritional profile of each of the protein source. Animal protein source is accompanied by the risk of high saturated fat and cholesterol content, which normally shouldn't be contained in a healthy diet (unless it is taken with little carbohydrate content). Plant protein sources, on the other hand, is low in fat and calories but does not contain as much protein as can be found animal sources. Animal protein can sometimes cause heart disease or even a stroke, in such a case you can easily make use of plant protein to achieve the desired nutritional benefit while not sacrificing your health. Whatever protein combination you decide to work with, just make sure that your diet has a low quantity of processed meat, but is rather rich in fish, egg, poultry meat, and dairy products, and also equally rich in plant protein such as fruits, legumes, and nuts. Don't focus on a single protein source; this will help you get a healthy balance of amino acids and other variety of nutrients present in both plant and animal protein sources.

CHAPTER FOUR

IMPORTANCE OF NUTS, SEEDS, AND FRUITS IN MAINTAINING A HEALTHY AND FIT BODY

Nuts and seeds are necessary because they can serve as a substitute for the conventional snack we are used to. Majority of the snacks we consume contain a variety of nutrients that will frustrate your goal of keeping a fit and healthy body. Cake for instance, even though is perfect as a snack (when you ignore the health risk it poses), has been prepared with a couple of unhealthy ingredients (most especially flour and sugar) that provide unhealthy calorie. If consumed as a snack, there is a high likelihood that it will disrupt your entire dietary goals. Nuts and seeds, on the other hand, are healthy foods which can be a source of protein and unsaturated fats. It has been discovered to protect against cardiovascular diseases, diabetes, and even helps to control body weight and lower the cholesterol content of the body. If consumed as a snack, you still get to enjoy the nutrients inherent in it, while not disrupting your laid down fitness goals. Fruits (dried) contain a large range of phytochemicals that help to promote your overall body health and boosts the body antioxidant capacity.

Eating nuts after a heavy workout session will also help provide enough protein and magnesium that aids relaxing and repairing of fatigued muscles, so the next time you're faced with the choice of consuming a healthy snack, instead of going for biscuits or some other snack, try out roasted nuts or dry fruits.

CHAPTER FIVE

THE RELATIONSHIP BETWEEN FLUIDS AND STAYING FIT

Without any doubt, fluids are one of the most important components of a healthy and successful diet. Whether you intend to lose, gain or maintain weight, the critical role played by water cannot be overemphasized. Fluid is an integral part of our body functions since it accounts for 75% of our body composition and is key in the transportation of nutrients in the body and the dispelling of waste from the body. Our body loses fluid as we go through our daily activities, and so to ensure the healthy functioning of our internal organs, the lost fluid has to be replaced either through various drinks or from the food we consume. People turn to refreshing beverages whenever they are dehydrated; nonetheless, water is considered as the best fluid restorer because it provides the necessary hydration, but without the unwanted calories. Majority of the energy drinks and beverages we turn to for hydration are electrolyte loaded and can be a source of needless calorie addition. However, the absence of calories inside water will make you feel full sooner, thereby aiding weight loss since you will eat less unnecessary calories from quick snacks. Water also helps to flush out waste from the body, an essential function that aids metabolism and weight loss.

Apart from water, the following fluids can also be taken to help with hydration, while also keeping us fit and healthy

a. **Coffee:** coffee is calorie free, and research has shown that the caffeine present inside a coffee can boost stamina and physical endurance levels. The coffee can be taken with milk but not with sugar, as the sugar is capable of negating the impact the caffeine is supposed to have.

b. **Fruit smoothies:** Homemade smoothies can be a healthy source of protein, fiber, vitamins, and minerals. Instead of choosing the option of prepackaged smoothies from the grocery store, you can meet up with your daily fruit recommendation for the day by making your own smoothies. You can leverage the health benefits of different fruits to stay fit and healthy. For instance, watermelon can help to soothe muscle soreness by the removal of lactic acid (a byproduct of exercise) at a high rate. It also contains amino acids in high content which help to increase blood flow, thereby decreasing the occurrence of muscle pains. Tomatoes contain lycopene, which helps to reduce damage to body tissues. Apple also is a good fruit snack that helps increase endurance levels as it contains quercetin which improves energy metabolism, thereby boosting endurance levels. Whatever fruit choice you stick with, ensure you achieve your goal of being hydrated, while also enjoying the nutritional benefits of a rich homemade smoothie.

CHAPTER SIX

RELATIONSHIP BETWEEN A HEALTHY SLEEPING HABIT AND STAYING FIT

The most effective diet and fitness routine need sufficient sleep to achieve the required results. This is because your sleep controls your diet. Research has shown that not getting enough sleep is capable of undoing the benefits of any healthy diet you take. Lack of sleep is also capable of increasing your craving for food. This is because the two hormones that control hunger (Leptin and Ghrelin) can be affected by sleep deprivation. Lack of sleep disrupts the hormones that regulate your appetite, increases your Ghrelin (appetite stimulator) levels, and reduces your Leptin (appetite suppressor) levels. Hence, studies have proven that people who suffer from sleep deprivation usually have a bigger appetite and tend to consume more calories, so if you intend to lose weight, sleep healthy.

It's also a known fact that the quality of sleep can also affect health status. Sleeping hours less than the required time increases your exposure to several health risks such as diabetes, heart disease, stroke, etc. So, if you desire to be fit and healthy, sleep.

CHAPTER SEVEN

ALTERNATIVES TO EXERCISE

Staying fit and healthy is not necessarily achieved by daily visits to the gym, or by a religious adherence to a fitness routine. You might be constrained by the high cost of registering for a fitness routine, or by a busy schedule such that it will be challenging to separate apart a time for a gym visit. If you desire to be fit, but you find yourself constrained by some factors such as budget or time, it shouldn't mark the end of your goal to stay fit and healthy. You might not be opportune to be registered in a gym, but you can still create a system that ensures you stay fit and healthy.

This is what has necessitated the incorporation of exercising into your lifestyle. You can plan your day to day activities in such a way that you can boost your metabolism and also be physically active. Take advantage of little activities such as avoiding the elevator and instead using the stairs, walking short distances, backpacking, mountaineering, engagement in sports, mowing your lawn, gardening, dancing, washing your car, etc. They are feasible and cheap alternatives to gym sessions that will provide you with arguably the same impact as going to the gym. If this is combined with a healthy diet and quality sleep time, your body goal is still on schedule to being achieved.

Fasting and Its Importance in Staying Fit

Over the years, fasting has gained popularity, most especially in the health community. This is because of the increasing knowledge of the various health benefits of fasting. Fasting is considered a safe route to weight loss since it limits calorie intake and boosts metabolism. You can try out the different types of fasting, and stick to the one which works for you, but you stand to reap enormous benefits if you are able to combine fasting with a nutritious diet.

CONCLUSION

A crucial element that should not be lacking if you will achieve your fitness goal is motivation. Following a diet will get boring at a particular time and emphasizes the importance of motivation. You can vary your diet from time to time if it will help you stay focused. Mix up the activities you do to exercise yourself so that your routine won't get boring. You can also work with like-minded people in order to keep you motivated every time you lose your motivation.

In conclusion, building and maintaining a healthy body isn't all about hitting the gym, or going through long hours of working out. Instead, it starts with a reorientation that fitness should not be a one-stop activity, but rather your lifestyle. Always work with the end of your goals in mind, as this is what will motivate you to keep up with the alien diet schedule that will deliver the sort of body you want

REFERENCES

https://m.onlymyhealth.com/why-important-stay-fit-healthy-1298540932

https://www.hhs.gov/fitness/eat-healthy/importance-of-good-nutrition/index.html

https://www.shape.com/healthy-eating/diet-tips/10-new-foods-power-your-workout

https://www.healthline.com/health/fitness-exercise-eating-healthy

https://thriveglobal.com/stories/10-simple-eating-habits-that-make-you-fit-and-healthy/

https://www.healthline.com/health/fitness-exercise-eating-healthy#carbohydrates

https://thriveglobal.com/stories/10-simple-eating-habits-that-make-you-fit-and-healthy/

https://www.telegraph.co.uk/health-fitness/nutrition/keeping-fit-what-to-eat-when-to-eat-and-why/

https://www.webmd.com/fitness-exercise/features/nutrition-tips-athletes

https://www.gaia.com/article/how-important-are-fats-healthy-diet

https://www.naturade.com/vegetable-protein-vs-animal-protein/

https://www.medicalnewstoday.com/articles/322827.php

https://www.healthline.com/nutrition/animal-vs-plant-protein#section5

https://www.disabled-world.com/fitness/nutrition/nuts-seeds/nuts-fruits.php

https://www.bustle.com/articles/161188-7-post-workout-foods-drinks-that-can-help-speed-up-recovery

https://www.acefitness.org/education-and-resources/lifestyle/blog/6675/healthy-hydration

https://www.everydayhealth.com/weight/the-importance-of-water-in-your-diet-plan.aspx

https://www.mensjournal.com/health-fitness/9-ways-to-get-fit-without-working-out-this-summer-w209040/golf-without-a-cart-w209048/

https://www.healthline.com/nutrition/fasting-benefits#section9

https://www.independent.co.uk/life-style/health-and-families/features/staying-motivated-to-achieve-your-fitness-goals-according-to-an-expert-a6813546.html